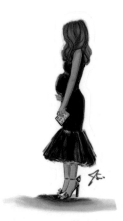

THE IVF PLANNER

A Personal Journal to Organize Your Journey through
In Vitro Fertilization (IVF) with Love and Positivity

MONICA BIVAS

BALBOA.
PRESS
A DIVISION OF HAY HOUSE

Balboa Press books may be ordered through booksellers or by contacting:

Balboa Press
A Division of Hay House
1663 Liberty Drive
Bloomington, IN 47403
www.balboapress.com
1 (877) 407-4847

Print information available on the last page.

ISBN: 978-1-9822-1325-1 (sc)
ISBN: 978-1-9822-1327-5 (hc)
ISBN: 978-1-9822-1326-8 (e)

Library of Congress Control Number: 2018911774

Balboa Press rev. date: 10/18/2018

Contents

To the memory of my baby daughter,
Isabelle Bivas (October 5, 2010)

PREFACE

The Journey of a Thousand Miles Starts with One Step

In vitro fertilization (IVF) has been a blessing in my life. However, it is also a roller-coaster ride of emotions, and with constant changes in the treatment itself, there is a lot of information to absorb. IVF treatments today are not the same as they were five, three, or even one year ago. Every day there is more and more research on fertility treatments to help those suffering from fertility issues, allowing not only for the greater possibility of getting pregnant but for having a healthy pregnancy and a healthy baby.

With IVF comes many emotions, including a sense of being overwhelmed and confused. My first three cycles were extremely stressful and difficult. My third IVF cycle ended with the stillbirth of my beautiful baby girl at thirty-nine weeks, three days before her expected due date. I did my fourth cycle almost immediately after my stillbirth, and even after having a big fat positive (BFP), I miscarried at seven weeks.

I realized that, in order to handle another round of IVF, I would have to take control of the situation based on what I'd lived through in previous cycles. To me, this meant knowing and accepting my medical situation. (I have double tube blockage caused by endometriosis. Even after a laparoscopy, they remain blocked.) I also have to know and accept my menstrual cycles, my body, my feelings, and my relationship with my partner.

After going through multiple cycles, I wanted to keep a record of my own IVF experiences. I bought an IVF journal already on the market, and G-d, it helped me so much! It helped me handle the stress and emotions of my cycle, focus on the process, and even nourish my relationship with my other half, my dear husband. I started to see my treatment in an objective way. I chose a different clinic and doctor, and I started to shift my thoughts, think more positively, and visualize my baby.

My last cycle actually resulted in my second baby. My first IVF cycle was also successful, culminating with the birth of my daughter, Eliyah, but I will share this story in my book about my personal journey through IVF.

With the help of my amazing husband, the clinic, and our medical team, I kept records and started to organize, track, and document all that was involved in the treatment. The journal helped me easily communicate with my reproductive endocrinologist (RE), nurses, and clinic. I was able to keep track of my questions and sometimes even find the answers myself as a result of tracking my IVF cycle.

After my third IVF cycle—and the subsequent birth of my stillborn daughter—I decided to do what I am doing now, coaching other women and couples who are about to begin IVF, already going through IVF, or in the latest of many cycles. Each of us suffering from fertility issues have different experiences, feelings, and emotions during the treatment. There is no way to know exactly how the various aspects of the treatment (medical, emotional, and psychological) will affect each individual.

However, having been through multiple cycles of IVF myself, I can offer you coaching on how best to approach the IVF process. I will help you create positive thought patterns, allowing you to see all the blessings and knowledge available to you and making your journey a joyful one. I know what you're going through because I have been through it too.

My main goal in creating this IVF journal is to add to the many positive experiences you can have during your fertility treatment.

In this book, I offer you guidance, valuable information, and advice to help you through each step of your treatment. I hope it helps you find focus, have a more organized approach to your treatment, and achieve better communication with your medical team, your partner, and even your own being, particularly if you decide to go through IVF by yourself.

I truly hope you will find relaxation, calm control, clarity, and connection with your own situation. It is also my hope that this journal will help you pass those long hours sitting in waiting rooms by keeping you focused on the positive and good things to come. I created this journal both as an information guide and opportunity for you to write your own story. One day when you have that rainbow baby, you can tell him/her/them the story of how they came into this world.

IVF women, we are made of courage and strength! We have been given this mission for a reason, and I have learned from my own experience that it is all worth it. Always remember the IVF journey, no matter the end result—negative, positive, or even cancelled cycles—takes strength and courage and teaches us to be disciplined. With all of that and an amazing amount of personal effort, the determination of your loved ones, and even the work of strangers who support you, this journey is definitely something to always feel proud of.

With all my heart and soul,

Monica Bivas

ACKNOWLEDGMENTS

Thirteen years ago, I was heartbroken when I discovered I have a fertility problem. After finding out my tubes were both blocked from endometriosis and after trying to unblock them with a laparoscopy was unsuccessful, my husband and I decided to go through IVF treatment so we could have a baby together.

During this time, my husband stood with me and was there as I cried. Although fear filled me, he told me that, no matter what or how much treatment cost, we would have a baby and I could count on it. Moshe Shai Bivas, baby, you are unique and supportive. I could not have done this without you. You are my rock, and I love you to infinity and beyond.

Amanda, Mom, you were also there for me even though you were not living here in the States. Your emotional and positive support were—and still is—beyond words. I love and trust you. I feel free with you, and besides being my mom, you are my best friend.

Eliyah, my first IVF baby, you were with me when we lost your baby sister, Isabelle, and when we went through treatment to have your little sister, Maya. Your love and understanding is beyond words. I love you!

Daniella, when I came into your dad's life, you were only a year and a half, but your pureness and beautiful soul opened my heart, prepared me for motherhood, and helped me decide to go on with my IVF journey. You were—and still are—like my own daughter, and you are a great sister to both Eliyah and Maya. I love you so much, and I am so grateful you came into my life!

To both my sisters, Sandra and Laura, even though you were far away, you were there for me all the time.

Finally, I want to thank everyone who supported me on my journey and helped me to get where I am, helping other women and couples have their dream baby and walk their journey in a positive way.

INTRODUCTION

How to Use Your Journal

IVF treatment is a complex process that can involve multiple medical teams and points of contact, and it is a significant financial investment. The cost for treatment includes numerous medications, appointments, daily tests, and procedures. Predictably, IVF is the theme of endless books, websites, blog posts, and articles.

I created this journal to help you organize the process, handle stress better, and bring focus and clarity to your personal journey. Yes, going through IVF brings on many strong and confusing emotions. It is challenging and expensive too, especially if insurance doesn't cover treatment, but using this book can ease all that stress and help you prepare for the path you have chosen. This journal can be used even if you are considering using donor eggs, a sperm and/or embryo donor, or a surrogate. The advice and most of the charts will still be applicable. You may need to make a few adjustments based on your specific needs.

I have organized this information based on what I found helpful during my procedures and with the feedback of other women. At the end of the day though, you are the one to decide how and how often to use this journal, which charts to use, and how to write in it. This journal shouldn't be a burden!

Before you start, I have some general suggestions for maintaining a positive attitude and managing your treatment: don't compare yourself to others. Every single woman going through IVF is different, and each cycle is different. What is normal for you might not be for other women. In IVF, there is no right or wrong.

Similarly, every reproductive endocrinologist (RE) and clinic is different. Your diagnosis and IVF experience depends on the clinic you choose. Your diagnosis will differ depending on the specialty of the RE, the cause of your infertility, and the number of times you have gone through IVF. However, as long as you are comfortable and receive kind, understanding care, all can go smoothly.

Prepare, but don't make plans based on an anticipated outcome. IVF has many variables. The timing of each step can change, and the outcome is not certain until the very end. What you can do, though, is prepare for the experience.

Get your information directly from the source. If you have any type of question, don't rely on Google or other medical personnel. You will receive conflicting information that will only confuse and overwhelm you. Your RE and his or her team should be able to answer any questions you have, relieve your doubts, and give you the advice you need. Never let information from insensitive or unverified sources confuse you. This will only bring you unnecessary stress.

IVF treatment options are continually evolving with new research and the discovery of new medicines. This is wonderful because it increases the possibility of a big fat positive (BFP) result and a healthy, full-term pregnancy. It can also affect how you interact with REs and clinics and your finances. This is why I've included a chart in this journal where you can record other treatment options, if need be.

Learn the basics of IVF treatment. This journal assumes that you have already decided that IVF is your only option or that you have done a cycle before. Similarly, it assumes that you have some basic knowledge of what an IVF cycle is. If not, part

I of this book and an online glossary, such as the one on the Society for Assisted Reproductive Technology's website (www. sart.org/Glossary), will help you to get started. In the back of the book, I have also provided a glossary of common IVF and online terms that you may run across during your IVF journey.

However, the best knowledge is a diagnosis and knowledge of your own situation. Why? There are multiple causes of infertility and many different types of treatment. Not all will apply to you. The diagnosis and treatment charts, with your RE's help, will help you organize and understand your situation better.

Know when enough is enough. Remember that IVF is a complex topic, so make sure you know when to put on the brakes. Too many details can make you feel not only overwhelmed, but cause an emotional firestorm even bigger than when you learned you would need to use IVF to have children. But remember, whether you are searching for more information or have realized that you have gone into enough detail, let your medical team know so they can help you.

Journal Overview

I have divided this IVF journal into eight parts. Each chapter starts with a detailed explanation on how to use the charts, logs, calendars, and journaling space. Because of all the emotional, psychological, financial, and physical considerations involved in IVF, my suggestion to you is to review each section and decide which ones are applicable to your situation before you start using your journal. But if you feel more confident jumping right in, go ahead and do it. This is your journey!

Part I: The Basics of IVF Treatment

This section outlines basic information about IVF treatment and the best way to prepare for it based on your diagnosis and situation. It describes each phase of the cycle, risks, and some of the general causes of infertility.

Part II: Medical Providers and Clinics

Part II provides a helpful outline for writing down information about the policies and procedures of IVF REs, clinics, pharmacies, and other medical providers. I recommend recording names, phone numbers, addresses, emails, and your medical provider policies for easy reference.

Part III: Finances

This section covers all the financial aspects of your IVF cycle: prices, payments, financing options, insurance coverage or noncoverage, taxes, and expense tracking.

Part IV: The IVF Cycle

In this section, charts are provided for managing the IVF cycle itself: the process, schedules, timing, medication record, egg retrieval (ER), embryo growth, and egg transfer (ET).

Part V: Your Wait Time and Results

This part is helpful for you to plan for and handle the end of the long IVF road, the two-week wait (2WW), and its results in a stress-free manner. It also comes with 14 coloring Mandalas, one for each day of the two-week wait (2WW), to help you ease your mind and creativity.

Part VI: Mind, Body, and Spiritual Support

This section is designed to help you plan your emotional and physical support during your IVF journey. Here you will find a chart that you can fill out by joining or creating a support group. It also helps you to explore the option of having therapy and assists you in handling your emotions through self-awareness.

Part VII: FET and Multiple Cycles

The journal is written for one cycle, but as we know, many women go through multiple cycles of IVF or opt for FET. This section offers some advice for longer-term treatments and space to record information about multiple cycles, making it easier to compare them later.

Part VIII: Glossary of Acronyms and Terms

This is a list of acronyms used throughout the book as well as a number of terms you might run across online in IVF groups or online comments. It is by no means an exhaustive list but can be used as a quick reference if you are unfamiliar with a term and what it means.

PART I
THE BASICS OF IVF TREATMENT

CHAPTER 1

THE BASICS OF IVF TREATMENT

The Struggle is Part of the Story.

—Anonymous

A basic understanding of the IVF process is crucial before you begin treatment.

In vitro fertilization (IVF) places a woman's egg and a man's sperm in a laboratory dish for the purpose of creating a viable embryo. The fertilized eggs become embryos, and then several, based on how many are viable, are placed in the woman's uterus, where they hopefully will implant.

Every cycle is different, but most follow a basic system. To be prepared for your specific situation, you must understand how the cycle works. I've divided the cycle into five phases to make it easier.

Precycle

This marks the beginning of your treatment, and it lasts a few weeks. Your body is being prepared for treatment, and you will have multiple appointments and tests at your clinic. You will receive schedules, instructions, medications, and so on from your RE and his or her team. Most women begin taking some medications in this phase.

A precycle includes some of the following tests and medications. A hysteroscopy and/or sonohysterography examines your uterine cavity for any issues. A semen analysis checks the quality, quantity, and motility of your partner's sperm. Both partners will be screened for infectious diseases, such as HIV/AIDS, hepatitis B and C, and chlamydia. Both will have to provide records from up-to-date physicals from their primary doctors. Some patients will take contraceptive pills during this phase to ensure their cycles will start at the right time or to regulate irregular cycles. Suppression medications are also given in this phase to ensure you do not ovulate too early. The RE will check your ovarian reserves to evaluate your egg supply. Some clinics use an follicle-stimulating hormone (FSH) or day 3 testing. It all depends on your RE and the clinic team. These tests, if they are performed, mark the close of the precycle phase.

Stimulation

This phase is all about egg production in the follicles. The main purpose of this phase is to stimulate the ovaries to produce multiple follicles or eggs instead of the single egg that is normally produced each month. This is necessary as not all eggs will be successfully fertilized. Retrieving more eggs increases the probability of having fertilized eggs. Keep in mind that fertilized eggs do not always develop normally, which is another reason for using multiple eggs.

During this phase, you will have regular transvaginal ultrasounds and blood work to check your hormone levels and ovaries. This part is also known as monitoring, which is done every other day. Based on the results of your monitoring tests, your RE will prescribe specific medications, adjusting them to your situation. You will also learn how many follicles are developing in each ovary. However, you must keep in mind that ultrasounds are not always accurate so there may not be a mature egg in each follicle. The exact number is known only after your egg retrieval.

Stimulation can last anything from a few days to two weeks. It is finalized with the trigger shot, a dose of medication given intramuscularly to induce ovulation and help the eggs to mature for fertilization. Your eggs will be retrieved between thirty-four and thirty-six hours after the trigger shot.

Egg Retrieval and Semen Collection

This is the procedural phase of IVF. Your RE will ask you to arrive at the clinic at a specific time and day for your egg retrieval. Most women are instructed not to eat or drink anything that morning. Other instructions may include not using perfume, deodorant, or scented lotions, which can interfere with lab procedures. Some clinics have a big team and allow your partner to be there during the procedure.

Additionally, many times it is not your RE who does the retrieval or transfer. This happens because clinics use work rotation schedules, especially when they have big medical teams. If you do not live close to the clinic, semen will be collected at the same site. However, if you live close, it can be collected at home and brought with you.

Once semen is collected, it is "washed," which means the sperm is separated from the seminal fluid and prepared for the fertilization process. Egg retrieval (also known as follicular aspiration) is a minor outpatient procedure during which the eggs are removed from your ovaries. Using ultrasound images for guidance, your RE inserts a very thin needle through the vagina and into the ovary. This needle is connected to a suction device that pulls the eggs out of the follicles one at each time. In most cases, an anesthesiologist provides intravenous medications so the patient sleeps through the procedure and doesn't feel a thing. You may experience some cramping and discomfort after the procedure, but this goes away within two days.

This procedure is done to both ovaries and only takes about thirty to thirty-five minutes. Once you are awake, your RE or nurse will tell you how many eggs were retrieved. After your eggs are retrieved, they are transferred to a lab and are kept in a warm environment similar to the environment in your fallopian tubes and uterus.

On the same day the eggs are retrieved, you will begin to take progesterone through either injections or vaginal or oral tablets, depending on your situation and your RE. Progesterone prepares your body for a possible pregnancy, helping the lining of the uterus get ready to receive the embryos.

Fertilization and Growth

After retrieval, your partner's semen and your eggs are placed together in a culture medium. A culture medium is a nutrient-rich substance that is used to cultivate microorganisms, providing ideal, specialized conditions for the egg and sperm and then resulting in the embryo. This is done with the hope that the sperm will enter and fertilize the eggs.

Depending on the quality, quantity, and mobility of the sperm, your RE may decide it is necessary to do an intracytoplasmic sperm injection (ICSI). Some patients also decide to do screening tests, such as a comparative genomic hybridization (CGH) and preimplantation genetic diagnosis (PGD).

Because these tests are expensive and not all clinics perform them, some patients decide not to do them. However, they are worth considering as they can help to find chromosomal abnormalities and diagnose previous causes of failed IVF. Assisted hatching is also recommended, depending on maternal age or previous failed IVF cycles. This is done before embryo transfer.

Embryo Transfer and Results

About three to five days after egg retrieval, depending on whether the patient used genetic testing, ICSI, or assisted hatching after fertilization, the embryos will be transferred to your uterus. A day 3 transfer means the embryo or embryos will be placed in the uterus after three days of growing in the lab; a day 5 transfer means they will grow in the lab for a total of five days.

The RE, clinic, and embryologists may change your transfer day, depending on how the embryo is growing. You might be set for a day 5 transfer, but if the embryologist determines that a day 3 transfer is preferable, your date will change.

On the transfer day, the most viable embryos are selected for transfer. The quality of embryos is usually determined by the number of cells an embryo has and how they fragment. Each clinic has its own grading system so this determination is very subjective. The Clinic Operations Chart in this journal has space for you to take notes about the grading system your RE and clinic team use.

When you arrive at your clinic for the transfer, your RE and embryologist will talk to you about the embryos' quality and the number to be transferred. Some clinics will even provide a picture of the embryos, which you can take home with you. Before the transfer, you might be given a mild sedative to help you relax. You will also be asked to drink water so your bladder will be full during transfer. Even though this is uncomfortable, it allows your RE to have the best access to the uterus.

A catheter is inserted through the vagina and cervix into the uterus, similar to an intrauterine insemination. Then a syringe containing the embryos is attached to the end of the catheter, and the embryos, cushioned by fluid, are pushed into the uterus. The waiting period after transfer depends on each clinic, but most will let you go after fifteen or twenty minutes of rest.

If you have extra embryos of a good quality, the clinic will offer to freeze them for transfer later. You will continue to take progesterone until the pregnancy test, which will be done ten to fourteen days after transfer and the HCG levels in your blood are measured. If the test comes back positive, it is repeated a few days later to see if levels of HCG are rising the way they are supposed to. You might be required to continue progesterone and any other support medications for a little longer.

Risks, Cancellations, and Possible Outcomes

Like any other medical treatment, IVF has some risks associated with it. The procedure may be canceled, even if it is already underway. My second IVF cycle was canceled because the dose I was told to inject myself with was too high. As a result, I got ovarian hyperstimulation syndrome (OHSS), which could be dangerous and even life threatening. Also the results of IVF are not always set in stone. A positive result on an IVF treatment does not always finish in a full-term pregnancy.

In this journal, the Clinic Operations Chart in chapter 3 will guide you through clinic-specific terms.

Risks

You can discuss these in detail with your RE and clinic team. IVF increases the risk of multiple-birth pregnancies, especially in women over thirty-seven years and when more than one embryo is transferred to the uterus at a time.

Fertility drugs can cause OHSS. When this happens, the ovaries become swollen and very painful as a result of developing too many follicles. You may experience bloating, vomiting, nausea, diarrhea, and abdominal pain. This may result in cancellation of your IVF cycle. It can last from a few days up to a week and can also be life threatening.

Cancellations

Here are some common causes for canceling an IVF cycle:

- Premature ovulation, when the egg is released before the egg retrieval date

- OHSS, which means that too many follicles develop at the same time

- An inadequate number of developing follicles

- Ovarian cysts, which can be detected before the treatment or develop during

Outcomes

An IVF cycle does not always end with a healthy, full-term baby. While that is well known, it is good to acknowledge all the potential outcomes so we are mentally prepared and ready to face unwelcome surprises. When a patient faces one of these situations, there is more waiting, testing, and decision-making. Your clinic and RE play an important role to help you through this part of the cycle. The best thing you can do to prepare is to be aware of all the possibilities—good and bad.

Miscarriage

Even if the pregnancy is developing normally and you have a confirmation ultrasound, a miscarriage (MC) can still happen. The chance of a miscarriage is 15 to 20 percent, which is the same as the chance of miscarriage in a natural conception.

Ectopic Pregnancy

This occurs when the embryo implants outside the uterus or in a fallopian tube. The percentage of women having an ectopic pregnancy with IVF is 2 percent.

Blighted Ovum

This is also known as an anembryonic pregnancy and occurs when the embryo attaches itself in the uterine wall and forms a pregnancy sac but does not develop.

Chemical Pregnancy

This is also common in natural conception and is actually a very early miscarriage, which takes place before anything can be seen on an ultrasound scan—usually around the fifth week of pregnancy. It means that, even though the embryo attached to the uterine wall, it failed to survive.

Some Causes of Infertility

Many factors cause infertility, and every patient who goes through IVF or any other fertility treatment is unique. Below you will find some causes of infertility, but if you need more information, please talk with your RE or medical team. There is also a list of organizations later on in this journal that you can refer to for more information.

Unexplained infertility happens in about 10 to 20 percent of patients, and there is no known cause. Health conditions like thyroid disease, cancer, celiac disease, and other diseases can also cause infertility.

Fallopian tube blockage or damage makes it extremely difficult or impossible for a fertilized egg to reach the uterus. Ovulation disorders, such as irregular ovulation or follicles failing to produce mature eggs, can cause infertility.

Endometriosis, a condition when uterine tissue grows outside of the uterus, affects the functionality of the uterus, fallopian tubes, and ovaries. Polycystic ovary syndrome (PCOS) is a common hormonal disorder that affects fertility in women of reproductive age.

Sperm issues, such as low production, reduced motility, or abnormalities in shape, can make it impossible for the sperm to fertilize the egg. Premature ovarian failure occurs when women before the age of forty lose normal ovarian function. This happens because the ovaries do not produce a normal amount of estrogen or release eggs on a regular cycle. Finally, uterine and ovarian fibroids and cysts, which can grow in the uterine wall, interfere with embryo implantation.

This is just a short list of possible causes of infertility, but the most important thing for you to do is understand your own diagnosis. When you learn about your condition and what options are available, you are more prepared for what will come.

This journal includes a Diagnosis Chart (chapter 2) for you to record your medical information and options.

CHAPTER 2

PREPARING FOR IVF TREATMENT

The difficulties of life are intended to make us better, not bitter.
—Anonymous

Your IVF journey can be a stressful road, a roller coaster of emotions and surprises. Even when things seem to be going perfectly, unexpected situations can arise. Here are a few tips on how to prepare for your IVF cycle and make the process smoother and more positive.

Understand Your Treatment Cycle

Not knowing what to expect can be stressful and make the treatment more difficult. The outcome of an IVF cycle is always unknown, so do not focus on the "what ifs" or your worries about it. Instead I suggest you focus on the treatment in a positive and calm way. How? Well, make your best effort to understand the treatment itself, your diagnosis, and all the possible outcomes before you even start. By doing this, you demystify your treatment and are more mentally prepared for any possible outcome.

Organize Your Time

IVF treatments generally follow a basic timeline, but they can still be unpredictable. Unexpected changes can create stress and uncertainty when they force you to alter your schedule. I recommend adopting a flexible mind-set so you are less bothered by unexpected changes.

Waiting is also something you must be prepared for. IVF involves a lot of time spent waiting, which can be very time consuming.

If you work, my suggestion is to give notice to your manager about your IVF treatment. If you don't work and are a housewife, organize your schedule so that you have flexibility.

Think About Your IVF as a Positive Journey, Not a Destination

IVF cycles are not quick treatments. There can be many months between finding out this is your only treatment option and the final conclusion of an IVF cycle. In some complicated cases, treatment can take years.

I am not saying this to scare you. I just want to prepare you in case your treatment takes longer than you expected. This is why I call it a journey. You can find more information about the success rates of IVF cycles at the Society for Assisted Reproductive Technology's website (www.sart.org).

Find a Network and Group Support

IVF is not an easy road. Sometimes we might find it difficult to share the journey with others—even with close family. But it's important to realize it is not healthy to walk this road alone, which is why I recommend joining or forming a support group of women who are also undergoing treatment. You have no idea how much a supportive group who know what you are going through can help. I have also seen many women build long-lasting friendships in the support group that I host. Facebook, Twitter, Instagram, and Pinterest are great sources for finding IVF and fertility support groups.

Using the Charts

The first charts in this journal cover your diagnosis information and IVF treatment plan. I suggest you complete the Diagnosis Chart ahead of time so you are less stressed about explaining your medical situation.

The Diagnosis Chart can be completed when you meet your RE, so make sure you ask for a detailed explanation of your diagnosis. Based on this, your RE will provide you with the necessary information and the plan he or she recommends. Make sure you take detailed notes of all he or she says.

After understanding the reasons why you need an IVF cycle, you can then start to fill out the Treatment Chart, which will help you understand the specifics of your plan. The Treatment Chart is easy to understand and is divided by boxes detailing the IVF phases. It ends with a box dedicated to the embryo transfer information. Here you can take notes about how your clinic grades the embryos and how many embryos will be transferred, based on your RE's recommendations.

Remember to ask questions about this process. For example, how many embryos will your RE recommend transferring at a time? (This is often based on your age.) How will that number affect the chances of success, and how high is the risk of multiple pregnancies?

When you finish completing these charts, you will have a good understanding of your diagnosis and will be ready to start your cycle.

DIAGNOSIS CHART

Summary of Diagnosis:

· Unexplained infertility (2018)

Treatment History:

3 IUI (Jun – Sept 2015)

D & C (April 2016)

HSG (Dec. 2016)

Biopsy (ERA = Receptiva DX)

1 Round Clomid (9/2017)

Recommended Treatment:

IVF

Treatment Chart

Protocol: _____

Planned Transfer Day: _____

Planned Procedures and Testing:

_____

_____

Phase 1 Notes:

_____

_____

Phase 2 Notes:

_____

_____

Phase 3 Notes:

_____

_____

Phase 4 Notes:

_____

_____

Phase 5 Notes:

_____

_____

Embryo Transfer Notes:

_____

_____

Journaling Space

_____

_____

_____

_____

_____

_____

_____

_____

_____

_____

_____

_____

_____

_____

_____

_____

_____

_____

_____

_____

_____

_____

PART II

MEDICAL PROVIDERS AND CLINICS

CHAPTER 3

YOUR MEDICAL TEAM

You are not Broken, you are breaking through.
—Anonymous

Once you choose a clinic and your RE, it is very important to understand your medical team's policies and procedures. Knowing how they operate, communicate, and interact with you and other patients can help eliminate surprises and minimize stress. You will also know who can answer your questions, where to look for answers, and what to expect during your cycle.

Using the Charts

Completing the charts in this chapter is very important. They should be filled out in the order they are provided. Start with the section about your clinic and its contact information. Don't be afraid to ask for the most important and specific contacts you will need. This is your cycle, and you are entitled to this information.

Next, fill out the Clinic Operations Chart. Every section in this chart corresponds with the main activities of the clinic and how it works. Be sure to fill out all the information or at least that which you consider most relevant to your specific situation.

The Clinic Affiliations Chart records the information of other medical groups that might be working with your clinic, such as the lab, pharmacy, obstetrician, and so on. Again, fill this out according to your situation and the information provided by your clinic.

The RE and Specialists Team Contact Chart is specifically designed for recording contact information for your RE and the team of specialists involved in your treatment cycle. It also includes your Personal Physicians and Specialists Chart. (Remember, you have your own doctors before starting this treatment, so I recommend you include their contact details in the journal as well).

Finally, there is a Questions Chart, which you can use to remember things you want to address at your next appointment. A journaling space is at the end to document information you received during your appointment or phone call and to record any thoughts or feelings you felt during the appointment or afterward.

CLINIC CONTACTS CHART

Contact: _MJ — Medical Assistant_

Phone: _858)720-3101_ Email: _mj@sdfertility.com_

Contact: _Dr. Brooke Friedman_

Phone:_____ Email: _SD Fertility Center_

Contact: _Shaylyn — Reception_

Phone:_____ Email: _____

Contact: _Mackenzie — Reception_

Phone:_____ Email: _____

Contact: _____

Phone:_____ Email: _____

Contact: _____

Phone:_____ Email: _____

Contact: _____

Phone:_____ Email: _____

Clinic Operations Chart

Orientation and Training Information:

_____

_____

_____

After-hours and Emergency Procedure:

_____

_____

_____

Requirements to Begin Cycle:

_____

_____

_____

Appointment Scheduling Information:

_____

_____

_____

Additional Testing Information:

_____

_____

_____

Clinic Operations Chart

Medication Information:

_____

_____

_____

Embryo Grading Information and Freezing Criteria:

_____

_____

_____

Cycle Completion and Cancellation Information:

_____

_____

_____

_____

Additional Information:

_____

_____

_____

_____

CLINIC AFFILIATIONS CHART

Organization: _____

Number:_____ Email: _____

Website: _____

Address:_____

Info/Policy/Hours: _____

Organization: _____

Number:_____ Email: _____

Website: _____

Address:_____

Info/Policy/Hours: _____

Organization: _____

Number:_____ Email: _____

Website: _____

Address:_____

Info/Policy/Hours: _____

Organization: _____

Number:_____ Email: _____

Website: _____

Address:_____

Info/Policy/Hours: _____

CLINIC AFFILIATIONS CHART

Organization: _____

Number:_____ Email: _____

Website: _____

Address:_____

Info/Policy/Hours: _____

Organization: _____

Number:_____ Email: _____

Website: _____

Address:_____

Info/Policy/Hours: _____

Organization: _____

Number:_____ Email: _____

Website: _____

Address:_____

Info/Policy/Hours: _____

Organization: _____

Number:_____ Email: _____

Website: _____

Address:_____

Info/Policy/Hours: _____

© 2018

RE and Specialist Team Contact Chart

RE: _____

Phone:_____ Emergency Phone:_____

Email: _____ Website: _____

Address:_____

Doctor: _____

Other: _____

Phone:_____ Emergency Phone:_____

Email: _____ Website: _____

Address:_____

Doctor: _____

Other: _____

Phone:_____ Emergency Phone:_____

Email: _____ Website: _____

Address:_____

Doctor: _____

Other: _____

Phone:_____ Emergency Phone:_____

Email: _____ Website: _____

Address:_____

Doctor: _____

Other: _____

RE and Specialist Team Contact Chart

Phone:_____ Emergency Phone:_____

Email: _____ Website: _____

Address:_____

Doctor: _____

Other: _____

Phone:_____ Emergency Phone:_____

Email: _____ Website: _____

Address:_____

Doctor: _____

OB-GYN: _____

Phone:_____ Emergency Phone:_____

Email: _____

Website: _____

Address:_____

Doctor: _____

Urology: _____

Phone:_____ Emergency Phone:_____

Email: _____

Website: _____

Address:_____

Questions Chart

Question:

Blood work for Immunology - Body
fighting off embryos?

Answer:

_____

_____

_____

Question:

_____

_____

Answer:

_____

_____

_____

Question:

_____

_____

Answer:

_____

_____

_____

QUESTIONS CHART

Question:

_____

_____

Answer:

_____

_____

_____

Question:

_____

_____

Answer:

_____

_____

_____

Question:

_____

_____

Answer:

_____

_____

_____

Journaling Space

_____

_____

_____

_____

_____

_____

_____

_____

_____

_____

_____

_____

_____

_____

_____

_____

_____

_____

_____

_____

_____

_____

_____

_____

_____

_____

_____

PART III

FINANCES

CHAPTER 4

IVF TREATMENT AND YOUR FINANCES

If you Stumble, make it part of the dance.

—Anonymous

Once you choose a clinic and your RE, it is very important to understand your medical team's financial policies and the estimated cost of your treatment. It is well-known that IVF treatment is not cheap, and it is very important to stay on top of the financial aspect of your treatment. Knowing how much and when you are required to pay will help you keep surprises and aggravation to a minimum.

Here in the United States, coverage of IVF treatment varies from state to state and is usually determined by your employer's insurance program. In Canada, IVF treatment may be covered by Medicare, which each province's health ministry governs. In the United Kingdom, a lottery system run by the National Healthcare System (NHS) determines coverage. Restrictions on coverage and the number of cycles you can receive depend on your medical condition and age and whether you have had IVF treatment in the past. Some countries in Europe offer complete coverage and others only partial, but the waiting lists can be long.

Using the Charts

The use of the charts in this chapter depends on whether you have insurance or not.

For Patients Who Have Insurance

The charts are based on insurance coverage in the United States. If you are outside the States, use the spaces that are applicable, and make adjustments as necessary. Remember, even if your insurance covers IVF, you will still need to thoroughly read your insurance policies. Most insurance plans have co-pays, payout limits, deductibles, and so on. Make sure you understand your insurance coverage before filling out the charts.

The Insurance Coverage Chart has three detailed sections to complete, including your insurance provider contact information, deductible amount, annual and lifetime spending limits, and the co-pay amounts for various services.

In the Coverage Details portion, you have the option to write in the number of IVF cycles your insurance covers. The second page of the chart has space for you to fill in your financial requirements and restrictions, which will assist you with creating a budget. The last segment helps you to track who pays your clinic and includes space for other providers such as pharmacies.

The Cycle Cost Chart and the Payment Tracking Chart will help you to determine exactly what your expenses are during the IVF process and how and when you will pay for them. It is important to find out how your clinic will bill you for your cycle. Ask whether they charge a set price or separately for each service, what procedures are included and which are not, if ICSI, PGD and other tests are included or are billed separately, and what other services you may be billed for.

Finally, use the Finance Notes Chart for any additional information you may find useful. Keeping a clear record of your payments ensures you will have all the necessary information in case questions arise regarding payments and finances. It can also help you forecast other upcoming expenses.

Insurance Coverage Chart

Insurance Provider Contact Information

Insurance Provider:_____

Member ID: _____

Number:_____ Emergency Number: _____

Website:_____ Email: _____

Web Login:_____ Web Password: _____

Coverage Details

Number of Cycles Included: _____

Annual Deductible:_____ Annual Max Spend: _____

Lifetime Max Spend: _____

Covered Services

Service:_____ Co-pay Amount: _____

Information: _____

Service: _____ Co-pay Amount: _____

Information: _____

Service: _____ Co-pay Amount: _____

Information: _____

Service: _____ Co-pay Amount: _____

Information: _____

Requirements for Coverage:

_____

_____

_____

Insurance Coverage Chart

Services Not Covered:

_____

_____

_____

_____

_____

_____

_____

_____

_____

_____

_____

_____

Payment, Referrals, Claims, and Reimbursements

Clinic Paid: _____

Payments Procedure: _____

_____

Referral Procedure: _____

RE Referral ID: _____

Primary Physician ID: _____

© 2018

Insurance Liaison Chart

Date:_____ Spoke To: _____ Reference Number: _____

Details:

_____

_____

_____

_____

_____

Date:_____ Spoke To: _____ Reference Number: _____

Details:

_____

_____

_____

_____

_____

Date:_____ Spoke To: _____ Reference Number: _____

Details:

_____

_____

_____

_____

Insurance Liaison Chart

Date:_____ Spoke To: _____ Reference Number: _____

Details:

_____

_____

_____

_____

_____

Cycle Cost Chart

Expense (e.g., Day 3 Testing)   Cost

_____   _____

_____   _____

_____   _____

_____   _____

_____   _____

_____   _____

_____   _____

_____   _____

_____   _____

_____   _____

_____   _____

_____   _____

_____   _____

_____   _____

_____   _____

_____   _____

_____   _____

_____   _____

_____   _____

_____   _____

_____   _____

_____   _____

_____   Total _____

PAYMENT TRACKING CHART

Vendor	Date	Invoice No	Amount

Finance Notes

CHAPTER 5

IVF TREATMENT AND TAXES: US CITIZENS GUIDE

My courage is stronger than my fear.

—Anonymous

Many women go through IVF and fertility treatments and are unaware that the cost of treatment may be tax deductible. Similarly, many women are aware but don't completely understand how to take advantage of the offer or simply don't do it. Because the possibility of tax deductions on fertility treatments like IVF, ultrasounds, medicines, and so forth exists, it is absolutely worthwhile to see if you are eligible and get back some of your hard-earned money.

As of October 2016, the IRS states you may deduct medical expenses that exceed 10 percent of your adjusted gross income (AGI) or 7.5 percent if you or your spouse is sixty-five years of age or older. Remember to check for the latest guidelines when doing your taxes. It can be confusing, but if you keep organized records of your medical expenses, you can quickly figure out whether your IVF cycle and other medical expenses are eligible for deduction or a tax refund.

If you have an accountant, I definitely recommend you pass this on to him or her. But if like most of us, you do not, you will have to prepare your taxes on your own and find out if you qualify for tax deductions.

How do you do this? Here are a few tips:

1. Know the rules. The IRS has many rules and very complicated restrictions and guidelines for taxes and deductions. Everything is based on your income level and the number of dependents you claim, and depending

on this, some medical situations can qualify. The IRS publishes an updated version of their tax guide every year. The portion you will need is Section 502, "Medical and Dental Expenses." It is a good idea to look this up to learn about these rules and guidelines. The IRS updates their publications frequently and offers detailed information on what expenses, income levels, dependents, and situations qualify for medical deductions. You can find this information at www.irs.gov/publications.

2. Add up all your qualified medical expenses for the year. Do not forget that you can include all your medical expenses, not only the ones related to your IVF cycle. Stay ahead of the game by keeping track of expenses and receipts before tax time. If you don't, you will have to track the information down, and this is time consuming. If you can't find the bills and receipts, try to find this information in your bank statements and canceled checks, or ask your providers to give you a copy of the receipts.

3. Determine your income level. When you complete your 1040 tax form and calculate your AGI, you can determine whether you are eligible to make medical expense deductions. Your AGI is your total income from taxable sources, minus allowable deductions like education expenses, contributions to IRAs or health savings or flexible spending accounts, and interest on student loans or mortgages.

4. Do your math. Once you determine your total medical expenses and your AGI, you can use these numbers to do your calculations. Take your time, and remember each situation is unique. Keep all the documents such as receipts, medical records, gas receipts, and so on to back up any deductions you take. If you don't have an accountant, you can find information and guidance at www.irs.gov. Make sure you have the latest information when preparing your taxes, as IRS publications are updated every year.

Using the Charts

To determine if your medical expenses qualify for deductions, you will need to calculate how much you spent on IVF and fertility-related medical expenses first. If you completed and used the Insurance and Cycle Cost and Payment Tracking Charts in chapter 4, you will have a good idea of your expenses already.

Use the space provided to make any necessary calculations.

Tax Calculations

_____

_____

_____

_____

_____

_____

_____

_____

_____

_____

_____

_____

_____

_____

_____

_____

_____

_____

_____

_____

PART IV
THE IVF CYCLE

CHAPTER 6

IVF CYCLE SCHEDULING

I accept the gift of life within myself.

—Anonymous

IVF is not an easy journey. There are many obstacles, and the process challenges us with many overwhelming feelings, emotions, and situations. The best thing we can do for ourselves is to mindfully shift our thought patterns and be conscious of our actions. How? By slowing down, listening to our mind and body, and practicing conscious self-care. Basically, just take it easy!

One of the many reasons IVF cycles sometimes fail to result in a healthy pregnancy is because of the stress and negativity we put ourselves through during the cycle. I know that "taking it easy"—particularly in a situation like IVF—is extremely hard (or sometimes impossible). But difficult circumstances like going through IVF are when we need to practice keeping a healthy mind-set more than ever.

An IVF cycle only lasts six to eight weeks, but it often feels like an eternity for us and our partners. This is why I highly recommend following the suggestions below to help you slow down and take it easy during your cycle:

1. Avoid taking on new, additional projects or extra obligations that may bring more stress into your life. Going through IVF treatment is a new project on its own and is stressful enough in addition to your regular activities, work, and home life. If you are unable to avoid taking on additional projects, try to set deadlines so you have plenty of time to concentrate on your cycle.

2. Set aside "me" time. Plan specific times for rest and self-care. Even if you feel like you don't need it, it is vital during your cycle. Believe me!
3. Commit to prioritizing your cycle. If you have other children or too many chores in your daily life, ask your partner to help you out a little more during this time. If you have family close to you, ask them for aid too. Some women do not like to talk about what they are going through because they feel ashamed, but IVF is not a thing to feel ashamed of! Any extra help you can get will be beneficial for you and will make your cycle easier.

Using the Charts

In this chapter, the charts focus on the timing and the schedule of your IVF cycle. Do not forget to review the Treatment Chart in chapter 2, the Clinic Operations Chart in chapter 3, and the IVF Basics in chapter 1 so you are familiar with the treatment phases of your cycle.

Remember that treatment dates can change, so be flexible when writing down your notes. If you need to make adjustments, go back and do so.

There are two charts in this chapter. The first is the Cycle Schedule Chart, where you can record which event marks the beginning of your cycle, the estimated date your cycle will begin, and the actual date when you begin treatment. It is helpful to record these dates for reference later, especially when you end up having multiple cycles. Your RE and your medical team should provide all of this information.

There is also journaling space for you to record any scheduling notes and your emotions, thoughts, or feelings about treatment.

Please don't forget that, as you fill your planner with IVF cycle dates, they are subject to change depending on treatment results and your own needs.

CYCLE SCHEDULE CHART

Event (e.g. Cycle Start)	Estimated Date	Actual Date

© 2018

Journaling Space

_____

_____

_____

_____

_____

_____

_____

_____

_____

_____

_____

_____

_____

_____

_____

_____

_____

_____

_____

_____

_____

_____

CHAPTER 7

THE CHERRY ON TOP: MEDICATIONS, STIMULATION, AND PROCEDURE

Be strong; you never know who you are inspiring.

—Anonymous

By this time, you may be taking some medications and have appointments, which means there is a lot going on with you and your cycle. You may also find yourself really overwhelmed by all the time you spend waiting, the number of appointments you have, and the almost daily blood tests required for your treatment.

However, it is critical that you indulge yourself a little during this time. Between all the blood tests, daily vaginal ultrasounds, and injections, try to squeeze in some time for a massage, or ask your partner to give you one. Watch a funny movie. One amazing, relaxing activity I found during my fifth round of IVF was coloring! Adult coloring books are an incredible, simple, and inexpensive tool to relax and open your mind using creativity.

Introducing positive rituals like meditation, yoga, painting, or anything else creative into your routine during IVF treatment will also make your cycle an easier one, adding that "cherry on top" during this difficult time.

Eventually though, you will see this treatment as an incredible blessing because it will bring you that rainbow baby you've always dreamed of.

Using the Charts

This chapter includes the Medication and Details Chart, where you should record which medications you are taking for your treatment. You will also find the Medication Log Chart. This form makes it easier to keep track of which medications you are taking and at which time of day. I've included several copies of this chart for your convenience.

You will also find the Stimulation Monitoring Notes and the Hormone Levels Chart for keeping track of your physical response to the treatment and medications. The Stimulation Monitoring Notes is divided into three parts. The first section is for tracking your stimulation activity. The second and third sections are for tracking follicle development in your right and left ovaries. Remember that some clinics do not provide this information unless you ask for it.

In the Hormone Levels Chart, record the date and your hormone levels at that time. I've included sections for the hormones most commonly tested for, but there are two additional subdivisions for other hormone tests.

Record information about your trigger shot and egg retrieval appointment information on the Egg Retrieval Planning Chart. The Egg Retrieval Results Chart is for recording details about how many follicles developed during your cycle, how many eggs were retrieved, and how many eggs were mature. It also has a space to record information about your partner's semen sample.

The Fertilization and Embryo Chart should be filled out with the information pertaining to your transfer date. The embryo transfer appointment usually occurs three to five days after your retrieval.

Finally, fill in the Embryo Transfer Chart with the main details of your transfer and the instructions for pre- and post-transfer.

MEDICATION DETAILS CHART

Medication: _____ Purpose: _____

Instructions for Use: _____

Medication: _____ Purpose: _____

Instructions for Use: _____

Medication: _____ Purpose: _____

Instructions for Use: _____

Medication: _____ Purpose: _____

Instructions for Use: _____

Medication: _____ Purpose: _____

Instructions for Use: _____

Medication: _____ Purpose: _____

Instructions for Use: _____

Medication: _____ Purpose: _____

Instructions for Use: _____

Medication Log

Date: _____

Cycle Day: _____

	M	T	W	Th	F	S
Su						
05:00						
06:00						
07:00						
08:00						
09:00						
10:00						
11:00						
12:00						
13:00						
14:00						
15:00						
16:00						
17:00						
18:00						
19:00						
20:00						
21:00						
22:00						

MEDICATION LOG

Date: _____

Cycle Day: _____

	M	T	W	Th	F	S
Su	____	____	____	____	____	____
05:00	____	____	____	____	____	____
06:00	____	____	____	____	____	____
07:00	____	____	____	____	____	____
08:00	____	____	____	____	____	____
09:00	____	____	____	____	____	____
10:00	____	____	____	____	____	____
11:00	____	____	____	____	____	____
12:00	____	____	____	____	____	____
13:00	____	____	____	____	____	____
14:00	____	____	____	____	____	____
15:00	____	____	____	____	____	____
16:00	____	____	____	____	____	____
17:00	____	____	____	____	____	____
18:00	____	____	____	____	____	____
19:00	____	____	____	____	____	____
20:00	____	____	____	____	____	____
21:00	____	____	____	____	____	____
22:00	____	____	____	____	____	____

MEDICATION LOG

Date: _____

Cycle Day: _____

	M	T	W	Th	F	S
Su						
05:00						
06:00						
07:00						
08:00						
09:00						
10:00						
11:00						
12:00						
13:00						
14:00						
15:00						
16:00						
17:00						
18:00						
19:00						
20:00						
21:00						
22:00						

MEDICATION LOG

Date: _____

Cycle Day: _____

	M	T	W	Th	F	S
Su	___	___	___	___	___	___
05:00	___	___	___	___	___	___
06:00	___	___	___	___	___	___
07:00	___	___	___	___	___	___
08:00	___	___	___	___	___	___
09:00	___	___	___	___	___	___
10:00	___	___	___	___	___	___
11:00	___	___	___	___	___	___
12:00	___	___	___	___	___	___
13:00	___	___	___	___	___	___
14:00	___	___	___	___	___	___
15:00	___	___	___	___	___	___
16:00	___	___	___	___	___	___
17:00	___	___	___	___	___	___
18:00	___	___	___	___	___	___
19:00	___	___	___	___	___	___
20:00	___	___	___	___	___	___
21:00	___	___	___	___	___	___
22:00	___	___	___	___	___	___

Medication Log

Date: _____

Cycle Day: _____

	M	T	W	Th	F	S
Su	___	___	___	___	___	___
05:00	___	___	___	___	___	___
06:00	___	___	___	___	___	___
07:00	___	___	___	___	___	___
08:00	___	___	___	___	___	___
09:00	___	___	___	___	___	___
10:00	___	___	___	___	___	___
11:00	___	___	___	___	___	___
12:00	___	___	___	___	___	___
13:00	___	___	___	___	___	___
14:00	___	___	___	___	___	___
15:00	___	___	___	___	___	___
16:00	___	___	___	___	___	___
17:00	___	___	___	___	___	___
18:00	___	___	___	___	___	___
19:00	___	___	___	___	___	___
20:00	___	___	___	___	___	___
21:00	___	___	___	___	___	___
22:00	___	___	___	___	___	___

Medication Log

Date: _____

Cycle Day: _____

	M	T	W	Th	F	S
Su	___	___	___	___	___	___
05:00	___	___	___	___	___	___
06:00	___	___	___	___	___	___
07:00	___	___	___	___	___	___
08:00	___	___	___	___	___	___
09:00	___	___	___	___	___	___
10:00	___	___	___	___	___	___
11:00	___	___	___	___	___	___
12:00	___	___	___	___	___	___
13:00	___	___	___	___	___	___
14:00	___	___	___	___	___	___
15:00	___	___	___	___	___	___
16:00	___	___	___	___	___	___
17:00	___	___	___	___	___	___
18:00	___	___	___	___	___	___
19:00	___	___	___	___	___	___
20:00	___	___	___	___	___	___
21:00	___	___	___	___	___	___
22:00	___	___	___	___	___	___

Medication Log

Date: _____

Cycle Day: _____

	M	T	W	Th	F	S
Su						
05:00						
06:00						
07:00						
08:00						
09:00						
10:00						
11:00						
12:00						
13:00						
14:00						
15:00						
16:00						
17:00						
18:00						
19:00						
20:00						
21:00						
22:00						

Medication Log

Date: _____

Cycle Day: _____

	M	T	W	Th	F	S
Su	___	___	___	___	___	___
05:00	___	___	___	___	___	___
06:00	___	___	___	___	___	___
07:00	___	___	___	___	___	___
08:00	___	___	___	___	___	___
09:00	___	___	___	___	___	___
10:00	___	___	___	___	___	___
11:00	___	___	___	___	___	___
12:00	___	___	___	___	___	___
13:00	___	___	___	___	___	___
14:00	___	___	___	___	___	___
15:00	___	___	___	___	___	___
16:00	___	___	___	___	___	___
17:00	___	___	___	___	___	___
18:00	___	___	___	___	___	___
19:00	___	___	___	___	___	___
20:00	___	___	___	___	___	___
21:00	___	___	___	___	___	___
22:00	___	___	___	___	___	___

MEDICATION LOG

Date: _____

Cycle Day: _____

	M	T	W	Th	F	S
Su	____	____	____	____	____	____
05:00	____	____	____	____	____	____
06:00	____	____	____	____	____	____
07:00	____	____	____	____	____	____
08:00	____	____	____	____	____	____
09:00	____	____	____	____	____	____
10:00	____	____	____	____	____	____
11:00	____	____	____	____	____	____
12:00	____	____	____	____	____	____
13:00	____	____	____	____	____	____
14:00	____	____	____	____	____	____
15:00	____	____	____	____	____	____
16:00	____	____	____	____	____	____
17:00	____	____	____	____	____	____
18:00	____	____	____	____	____	____
19:00	____	____	____	____	____	____
20:00	____	____	____	____	____	____
21:00	____	____	____	____	____	____
22:00	____	____	____	____	____	____

MEDICATION LOG

Date: _____

Cycle Day: _____

	M	T	W	Th	F	S
Su	___	___	___	___	___	___
05:00	___	___	___	___	___	___
06:00	___	___	___	___	___	___
07:00	___	___	___	___	___	___
08:00	___	___	___	___	___	___
09:00	___	___	___	___	___	___
10:00	___	___	___	___	___	___
11:00	___	___	___	___	___	___
12:00	___	___	___	___	___	___
13:00	___	___	___	___	___	___
14:00	___	___	___	___	___	___
15:00	___	___	___	___	___	___
16:00	___	___	___	___	___	___
17:00	___	___	___	___	___	___
18:00	___	___	___	___	___	___
19:00	___	___	___	___	___	___
20:00	___	___	___	___	___	___
21:00	___	___	___	___	___	___
22:00	___	___	___	___	___	___

Medication Log

Date: _____

Cycle Day: _____

	M	T	W	Th	F	S
Su						
05:00						
06:00						
07:00						
08:00						
09:00						
10:00						
11:00						
12:00						
13:00						
14:00						
15:00						
16:00						
17:00						
18:00						
19:00						
20:00						
21:00						
22:00						

MEDICATION LOG

Date: _____

Cycle Day: _____

	M	T	W	Th	F	S
Su	___	___	___	___	___	___
05:00	___	___	___	___	___	___
06:00	___	___	___	___	___	___
07:00	___	___	___	___	___	___
08:00	___	___	___	___	___	___
09:00	___	___	___	___	___	___
10:00	___	___	___	___	___	___
11:00	___	___	___	___	___	___
12:00	___	___	___	___	___	___
13:00	___	___	___	___	___	___
14:00	___	___	___	___	___	___
15:00	___	___	___	___	___	___
16:00	___	___	___	___	___	___
17:00	___	___	___	___	___	___
18:00	___	___	___	___	___	___
19:00	___	___	___	___	___	___
20:00	___	___	___	___	___	___
21:00	___	___	___	___	___	___
22:00	___	___	___	___	___	___

Stimulation Monitoring Notes

Stimulation Monitoring Overview:

_____

_____

_____

_____

_____

_____

Right Ovary Notes:

_____

_____

_____

_____

_____

_____

Left Ovary Notes:

_____

_____

_____

_____

_____

_____

Hormone Levels Chart

Estradiol:

_____

_____

_____

Progesterone:

_____

_____

_____

LH:

_____

_____

_____

FSH:

_____

_____

_____

Other: _____

_____

_____

© 2018

_____

_____

Other:

_____

_____

_____

Egg Retrieval Planning Chart

Trigger Shot Information:

_____

_____

_____

Egg Retrieval Information:

_____

_____

_____

Retrieval Day Instruction:

_____

_____

_____

Semen Sample Instruction:

_____

_____

_____

Post-Retrieval Plan:

_____

_____

_____

Notes:

_____

_____

_____

_____

Egg Retrieval Results Chart

Egg Retrieval Information:

_____

_____

_____

_____

_____

_____

_____

_____

Semen Sample Information:

_____

_____

_____

_____

_____

_____

_____

_____

_____

EGG RETRIEVAL GROWTH CHART

Number of Eggs Fertilized: _____

Number w/ICSI:_____

Embryo Growth Information

Date: _____ Cycle Day: _____ No. of Embryos: _____

Notes:

_____

_____

Date: _____ Cycle Day: _____ No. of Embryos: _____

Notes:

_____

_____

Date: _____ Cycle Day: _____ No. of Embryos: _____

Notes:

_____

_____

Date: _____ Cycle Day: _____ No. of Embryos: _____

Notes:

_____

_____

Embryo Transfer Chart

Embryo Transfer Information:

3 Day Transfer ☐   5 Day Transfer ☐   Other ☐

Transfer Day Instructions:

_____

_____

Date:_____ Cycle Day: _____ No. of Embryos: _____

Notes:

_____

_____

Post-Transfer Instructions:

_____

_____

Transfer Results:

No. of Embryos Available: ____ No. of Embryos Transferred: ____

Embryo 1:

_____

_____

Embryo 2:

_____

_____

Embryo 3:

_____

_____

Embryo 4:

_____

_____

PART V

YOUR WAIT TIME AND RESULTS

CHAPTER 8

THE TWO-WEEK WAIT (2WW)

I allow new beginnings in my life.

—Anonymous

Here we are at the two-week wait (2WW)! This is the time period between the embryo transfer and your pregnancy test at the clinic. In my opinion, this is the most difficult part of an IVF cycle, and you can trust me: I have been there five times! The 2WW seems to last forever. The days pass by so slowly.

In most cases, the 2WW is between nine and twelve days. Try your best to relax and focus on positive thoughts and healthy activities. In case you are short on ideas, I've included a list of activities that I enjoyed, as well as 14 coloring mandalas to ease your mind and wake up your creativity. I suggest brainstorming with your partner and making a list of things that you like to do too!

♦ Read self-help and positive mind-set books. I loved visiting the Hay House website (www.hayhouse.com). They have many wonderful books and journals to help you stay positive and make yourself a happy lady!

♦ Clean up. Organize your clothes, closets, basement, and anywhere else in your house that could use some attention. Or rearrange a room. Be gentle with yourself, of course! This was an awesome activity. I loved it!

♦ If you can afford it, have a getaway weekend with your partner. I found that natural, historical, or cultural places were good destinations. We visited a beautiful Amish village, and I especially loved the cute antique stores.

♦ Cook delicious recipes and be creative in the kitchen.

♦ As I mentioned before, work on adult coloring books. They are amazing. That was one of my favorite activities.

♦ Watch romance and comedy movies. I did that a lot with my partner.

Learn to knit! If you already know how, then make something simple like a scarf. This also helps pass the time faster.

Using the Charts

In this chapter, use the 2WW Calendar Chart to plan activities on a daily basis to help you pass the time between your embryo transfer and test. The 2WW Notes section is provided for recording any testing notes from your RE or clinic or any over-the-counter pregnancy tests that you may take. (Personally, I did not want to put more pressure and stress on myself and did not use any pregnancy test at home in case it was negative.)

Embryo implantation can occur at different times and depends on many factors. Because of all this, I chose to wait until the beta test with my clinic. But again, this is your cycle, and it is your choice whether to do a home pregnancy test or not.

2WW Calendar Chart

Wait Day 1:

_____

_____

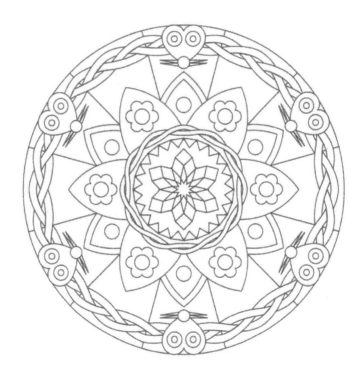

2WW Calendar Chart

Wait Day 2:

_____

_____

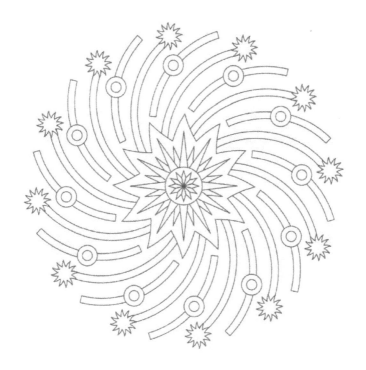

2WW Calendar Chart

Wait Day 3:

_____

_____

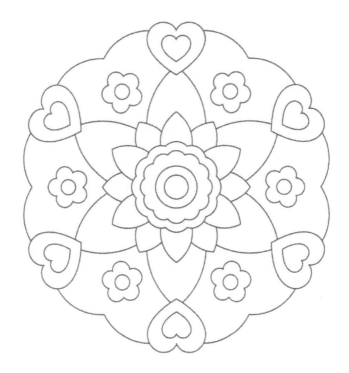

2WW Calendar Chart

Wait Day 4:

_____

_____

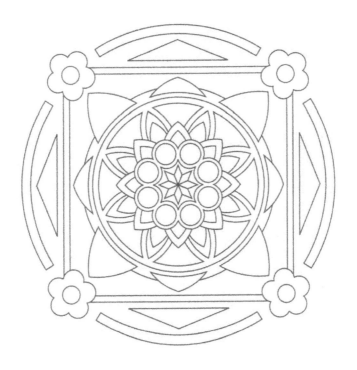

2WW Calendar Chart

Wait Day 5:

_____

_____

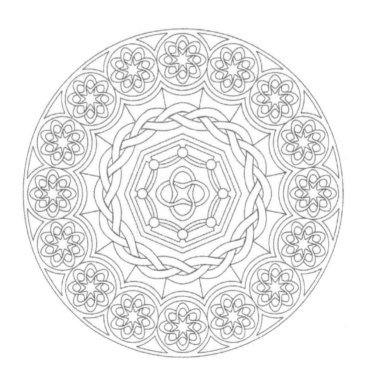

2WW Calendar Chart

Wait Day 6:

_____

_____

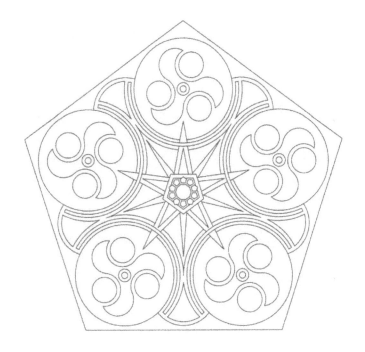

2WW Calendar Chart

Wait Day 7:

_____

_____

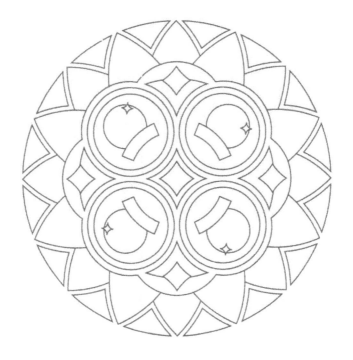

2WW Calendar Chart

Wait Day 8:

_____

_____

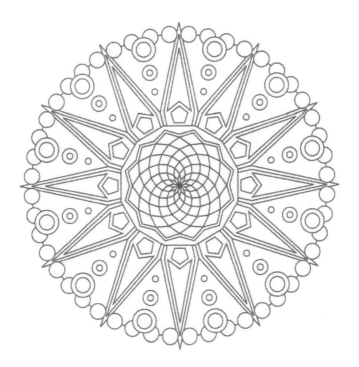

2WW Calendar Chart

Wait Day 9:

_____

_____

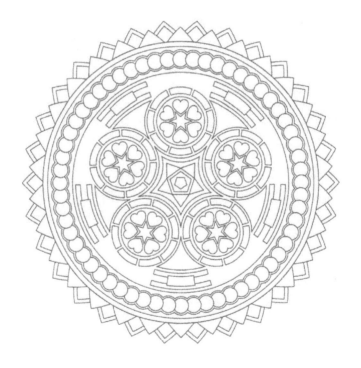

2WW Calendar Chart

Wait Day 10:

_____

_____

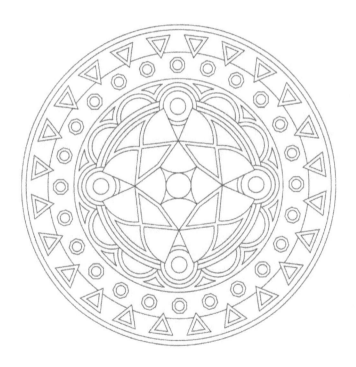

© 2018

2WW Calendar Chart

Wait Day 11:

_____

_____

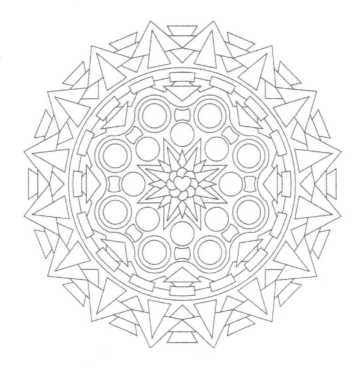

2WW Calendar Chart

Wait Day 12:

_____

_____

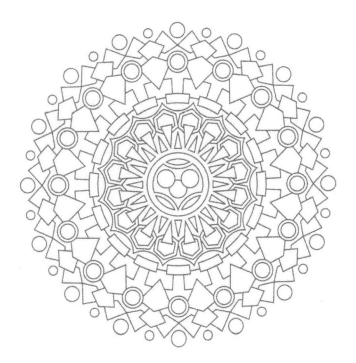

2WW Calendar Chart

Wait Day 13:

_____

_____

© 2018

2WW Calendar Chart

Wait Day 14:

_____

_____

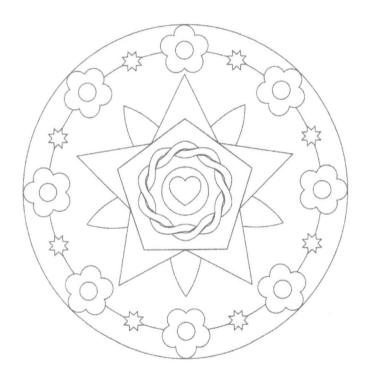

2WW Notes

CHAPTER 9

PREPARING FOR YOUR RESULTS

It only takes one. Try to stay Positive.

—Anonymous

We are now close to the end of your 2WW, which probably felt like the longest two weeks of your life! The reality we need to prepare for is that not all IVF cycles work. Success rates depend on many factors like age, clinic, treatment, diagnosis, and so on, but even under the best conditions, the cycle can end in a big fat negative (BFN). This is why—while it is important to remain hopeful, positive, and excited—we also need a plan B in case the results are negative.

A fallback plan cannot take away the pain of having a negative result, but it can help you to get through that hard time if it comes.

Using the Charts

The first chart is the Pregnancy Test Prepping Chart. This chart is for keeping track of the results of your IVF pregnancy tests, also known as beta tests. These beta tests measure the amount of HCG in your blood, which the placenta produces shortly after the embryo implants in the uterine lining.

To fill out this form, ask your clinic team for information about pre-testing instructions, which hormones are tested, what levels are considered desirable, and what the general testing procedure is. Some clinics perform only one test; others perform a two-day test. Ask your RE what qualifies as a positive result and what is considered a negative result. The next two charts are for compiling post-test results and options for possible test outcomes. One chart is for a BFP; the other is for a BFN.

Remember, even after a positive pregnancy result, some IVF pregnancies end due to unforeseen circumstances, like an ectopic pregnancy or failure to implant. If your results are negative, think again about your fertility options and discuss them with your partner. Decide what to do next. Perhaps you want to take a break before starting another cycle, or maybe your insurance covers more than one cycle in a row, and you can go ahead and do another one.

Look for group support. (You can find some great fertility groups online. You can join mine here: www.facebook.com/groups/theivfjourney.) Also check my website to see the services I offer at www.monicabivas.com. I offer support and coaching before, during, and after your cycle. I have been there, and I know exactly how you feel.

Finally, in chapter 12 there is more space to organize your notes for personal and group support. If you have a positive outcome, congratulations! I am also here to support you and guide you!

Pregnancy Test Prep Chart

Test Date: _____ Test Time: _____

Prep Notes:

_____

_____

_____

_____

_____

_____

_____

_____

_____

_____

_____

_____

_____

_____

_____

_____

_____

_____

BFN Chart

Emotional Support Resources and Plans:

_____

_____

_____

_____

_____

_____

_____

_____

Fertility Options Moving Forward:

_____

_____

_____

_____

_____

_____

_____

_____

BFP Chart

Pregnancy Announcement Plans:

_____

_____

_____

_____

Post-positive Test Notes:

_____

_____

_____

_____

Post-positive Medication Notes:

_____

_____

_____

_____

Release to OB-GYN Notes:

_____

_____

_____

_____

CHAPTER 10

DEALING WITH THE RESULTS

In Chaos there is Fertility.

—Anonymous

If you are facing the disappointment of a negative result, know my heart is with you. No words, no sorry, and no condolences exist for a failed cycle, but please know that every negative situation in life does ease with time and the pain will not be there in your mind and heart forever.

Besides the emotional pain, you are probably also feeling physically exhausted from all the hormones and medications that are still in your body, so you may experience mood swings and sadness. Make sure you rely on friends and family for support and comfort. Do not go through this alone! Or talk with friends in the support groups you are a member of.

My advice is for you to focus on yourself and your healing. Trust me. My third IVF cycle was positive, and I experienced a healthy pregnancy all the way to my thirty-ninth week. Everything seemed normal, but three days before my due date, my baby girl died in my womb because of a blood clot in her umbilical cord. It was not easy, but the pain didn't last forever. We must go on in life.

If this were your first IVF cycle, you might find comfort in knowing that the first time often is like a trial run and is not as successful as expected. Even for women without fertility issues, Mother Nature only has about a 25 percent success rate.

Using the Charts

Use the BFN Follow-up Chart during your follow-up appointment after the negative result. Fill it out with all the information you get at this appointment and keep it for your records in case you decide to go for another IVF cycle.

If you got a BFP, congratulations! You deserve this! This chapter also includes a BFP Follow-up Chart. Follow the same steps to fill it out when you go to your follow-up appointment after getting your results. If all goes well, you will be transferred from your RE and your clinic to your OB-GYN sometime during your first trimester. Don't forget that the end of this road is just the beginning of another one. You should continue to empower yourself during your pregnancy and motherhood, exactly the same way you did during your IVF cycle. Enjoy your time and your pregnancy!

BFN Follow-up Chart

Appointment Details:

_____

_____

Cycle Review Notes:

_____

_____

_____

_____

Possible Reasons for Failed Cycle:

_____

_____

_____

_____

Options for Moving Forward:

_____

_____

_____

_____

BFP Follow-up Chart

Appointment Details:

_____

_____

Cycle Review Notes:

_____

_____

_____

_____

_____

_____

_____

_____

_____

_____

_____

_____

_____

_____

_____

_____

PART VI

MIND, BODY, AND SPIRITUAL SUPPORT

CHAPTER 11

SURVIVING THE IVF EMOTIONAL ROLLER COASTER

Forget all the reasons why it won't work and
believe the one reason why it will.

—Anonymous

IVF is often compared to an emotional roller-coaster ride because of the many ups and downs during the treatment. There is a mix of feelings: hope, excitement, disappointment, sadness, loss, joy, stress, exhaustion, determination, and many others.

It's a crazy experience that can even make the strongest woman spin. As I've mentioned before, the best way to handle this ride is by practicing self-awareness, meditation, yoga, and any other positive activity that helps you shift your thoughts and actions. By default, this eases your emotions, helping you focus and stay more relaxed.

I also suggest writing about your journey. Journaling, a great tool to develop self-awareness, provides you with a clear record of past events. And it is a safe and easy way to reduce stress. If you journal already, then it makes the treatment process easier. If you are new to journaling, I suggest finding a nice notebook and a pen or pencil you enjoy writing with and start right away. Journaling helps you to clarify your thoughts, behaviors, emotions, desires, needs, and feelings and strengthens your sense of self.

Using the Charts

The journaling space in this chapter will help you to practice self-awareness by writing about your emotions and thoughts during your IVF cycle. Use it as often as you want. There is no specific time frame for it. This chart can provide great insight on how you can handle your ups and downs during the cycle.

The IVF Cycle Advice Chart gives you a place to write down any advice you've received before, during, and after your cycle. Reviewing this information can help you decide whether to go through IVF treatment again, regardless of whether you got a positive result or not.

Journaling Space

Date: _____

Mood: _____

Thoughts/Feelings/Notes:

_____

_____

_____

_____

_____

_____

_____

_____

Date: _____

Mood: _____

Thoughts/Feelings/Notes:

_____

_____

_____

_____

_____

_____

_____

_____

Journaling Space

Date: _____

Mood: _____

Thoughts/Feelings/Notes:

_____

_____

_____

_____

_____

_____

_____

_____

Date: _____

Mood: _____

Thoughts/Feelings/Notes:

_____

_____

_____

_____

_____

_____

_____

_____

Journaling Space

Date: _____

Mood: _____

Thoughts/Feelings/Notes:

_____

_____

_____

_____

_____

_____

_____

_____

Date: _____

Mood: _____

Thoughts/Feelings/Notes:

_____

_____

_____

_____

_____

_____

_____

_____

Journaling Space

Date: _____

Mood: _____

Thoughts/Feelings/Notes:

_____

_____

_____

_____

_____

_____

_____

_____

Date: _____

Mood: _____

Thoughts/Feelings/Notes:

_____

_____

_____

_____

_____

_____

_____

_____

Journaling Space

Date: _____

Mood: _____

Thoughts/Feelings/Notes:

_____

_____

_____

_____

_____

_____

_____

_____

Date: _____

Mood: _____

Thoughts/Feelings/Notes:

_____

_____

_____

_____

_____

_____

_____

_____

© 2018

Journaling Space

Date: _____

Mood: _____

Thoughts/Feelings/Notes:

_____

_____

_____

_____

_____

_____

_____

_____

Date: _____

Mood: _____

Thoughts/Feelings/Notes:

_____

_____

_____

_____

_____

_____

_____

_____

Journaling Space

Date: _____

Mood: _____

Thoughts/Feelings/Notes:

_____

_____

_____

_____

_____

_____

_____

_____

Date: _____

Mood: _____

Thoughts/Feelings/Notes:

_____

_____

_____

_____

_____

_____

_____

_____

Journaling Space

Date: _____

Mood: _____

Thoughts/Feelings/Notes:

_____

_____

_____

_____

_____

_____

_____

_____

Date: _____

Mood: _____

Thoughts/Feelings/Notes:

_____

_____

_____

_____

_____

_____

_____

_____

Journaling Space

Date: _____

Mood: _____

Thoughts/Feelings/Notes:

_____

_____

_____

_____

_____

_____

_____

_____

Date: _____

Mood: _____

Thoughts/Feelings/Notes:

_____

_____

_____

_____

_____

_____

_____

_____

Journaling Space

Date: _____

Mood: _____

Thoughts/Feelings/Notes:

_____

_____

_____

_____

_____

_____

_____

_____

_____

Date: _____

Mood: _____

Thoughts/Feelings/Notes:

_____

_____

_____

_____

_____

_____

_____

_____

_____

© 2018

JOURNALING SPACE

Date: _____

Mood: _____

Thoughts/Feelings/Notes:

_____

_____

_____

_____

_____

_____

_____

_____

Date: _____

Mood: _____

Thoughts/Feelings/Notes:

_____

_____

_____

_____

_____

_____

_____

_____

Journaling Space

Date: _____

Mood: _____

Thoughts/Feelings/Notes:

_____

_____

_____

_____

_____

_____

_____

Date: _____

Mood: _____

Thoughts/Feelings/Notes:

_____

_____

_____

_____

_____

_____

_____

IVF Cycle Advice Chart

Source: _____

Tip:

_____

_____

_____

_____

_____

Source: _____

Tip:

_____

_____

_____

_____

_____

Source: _____

Tip:

_____

_____

_____

_____

_____

IVF Cycle Advice Chart

Source: _____

Tip:

_____

_____

_____

_____

_____

Source: _____

Tip:

_____

_____

_____

_____

_____

Source: _____

Tip:

_____

_____

_____

_____

_____

CHAPTER 12

GATHERING YOUR SUPPORT NETWORK

Make a point to show yourself compassion. You are worthy.

—Anonymous

There are several ways to build your support network. One method is by searching for support groups on social media channels. I personally like this method the best because you can interact with women from all over the world and exchange tips, ideas, and support that helps you handle your cycle's ups and downs and results. Remember that you are always welcome in my group too (www.facebook.com/groups/theivfjourney). You can also find one-on-one coaching options through my website (www.monicabivas.com).

Another option to build your network is checking out nonprofit and fertility organizations, such as the Society for Assisted Reproductive Technology (www.sart.org), the American Fertility Association (www.theafa.org), the American Society for Reproductive Medicine and Resolve (www.asrm.org), and the National Infertility Organization (www.resolve.org). Search and take note of the ones that you identify with most. Some offer free fertility resources and have free groups you can join and mailing lists that send information about IVF treatment.

Also remember you can get support from your friends, family, mentors, and other women you meet who are going through or have undergone IVF cycles. You may find it helpful to find a therapist as you go through your IVF journey. And finally, you might find support from books or websites.

Using the Charts

In this chapter, there are two charts. The Support Network Chart is for tracking your personal support network, like therapists, social media groups, local groups, and specific people. You can also make a list of your favorite support resources, such as websites, books, or online groups in the Support Resource Chart.

SUPPORT NETWORK CHART

Source of Support: _____

Details:

_____

_____

_____

Source of Support: _____

Details:

_____

_____

_____

Source of Support: _____

Details:

_____

_____

_____

Source of Support: _____

Details:

_____

_____

_____

Support Network Chart

Source of Support: _____

Details:

_____

_____

_____

Source of Support: _____

Details:

_____

_____

_____

Source of Support: _____

Details:

_____

_____

_____

Source of Support: _____

Details:

_____

_____

_____

Support Resource Chart

Resource: _____

Details:

_____

_____

Resource: _____

Details:

_____

_____

Resource: _____

Details:

_____

_____

Resource: _____

Details:

_____

_____

Resource: _____

Details:

_____

_____

PART VII

FET AND MULTIPLE CYCLES

CHAPTER 13

FET AND MULTIPLE CYCLES

Believe that you will succeed and you will.

—Anonymous

When we face two, three, four, or even more IVF cycles, we can get overwhelmed and start focusing on the negative more than the positive. Try to find the good things to focus on in your situation instead. For example, if you've had a BFP in a previous cycle and are hoping for a sibling for the IVF baby you already have, focus on the positive: you already have one miracle baby.

Using the Charts

No matter what you choose to do, whether you decide to go ahead and start another cycle immediately or take some time for you and your partner, this journal will adapt to your decision. In this chapter, you will find a Post-Cycle Review Chart where you can summarize each cycle and compare it to your previous cycles.

You will also find a Multiple Cycle journaling space for writing notes and suggestions based on previous cycles, feelings about that particular cycle, and personal plans for the next cycle. Both these charts are intended to help you evaluate and understand how each cycle went and make your current cycle easier and more understandable.

Post-Cycle Review Chart

Cycle Number: _____ Cycle Date: _____ Protocol: _____

General Summary:

_____

_____

Medication Summary:

_____

_____

Stimulation Results Summary:

_____

_____

RE Response:

_____

_____

Protocol Recommendation for Future Cycles:

_____

_____

Post-Cycle Testing Recommendations and Results:

_____

_____

MULTIPLE CYCLE JOURNALING SPACE

Cycle Number: _____ Cycle Date: _____

Notes:

_____

_____

_____

_____

_____

_____

_____

_____

_____

_____

_____

_____

_____

_____

_____

_____

_____

_____

_____

_____

_____

POST-CYCLE REVIEW CHART

Cycle Number: _____ Cycle Date: _____ Protocol: _____

General Summary:

_____

_____

Medication Summary:

_____

_____

Stimulation Results Summary:

_____

_____

RE Response:

_____

_____

Protocol Recommendation for Future Cycles:

_____

_____

Post-Cycle Testing Recommendations and Results:

_____

_____

© 2018

Multiple Cycle Journaling Space

Cycle Number: _____ Cycle Date: _____

Notes:

_____

_____

_____

_____

_____

_____

_____

_____

_____

_____

_____

_____

_____

_____

_____

_____

_____

_____

_____

_____

_____

_____

© 2018

Post-Cycle Review Chart

Cycle Number: _____ Cycle Date: _____ Protocol: _____

General Summary:

_____

_____

Medication Summary:

_____

_____

Stimulation Results Summary:

_____

_____

RE Response:

_____

_____

Protocol Recommendation for Future Cycles:

_____

_____

Post-Cycle Testing Recommendations and Results:

_____

_____

MULTIPLE CYCLE JOURNALING SPACE

Cycle Number: _____ Cycle Date: _____

Notes:

_____

_____

_____

_____

_____

_____

_____

_____

_____

_____

_____

_____

_____

_____

_____

_____

_____

_____

_____

_____

_____

Post-Cycle Review Chart

Cycle Number: _____ Cycle Date: _____ Protocol: _____

General Summary:

_____

_____

Medication Summary:

_____

_____

Stimulation Results Summary:

_____

_____

RE Response:

_____

_____

Protocol Recommendation for Future Cycles:

_____

_____

Post-Cycle Testing Recommendations and Results:

_____

_____

© 2018

Multiple Cycle Journaling Space

Cycle Number: _____ Cycle Date: _____

Notes:

_____

_____

_____

_____

_____

_____

_____

_____

_____

_____

_____

_____

_____

_____

_____

_____

_____

_____

_____

_____

_____

_____

Post-Cycle Review Chart

Cycle Number: _____ Cycle Date: _____ Protocol: _____

General Summary:

_____

_____

Medication Summary:

_____

_____

Stimulation Results Summary:

_____

_____

RE Response:

_____

_____

Protocol Recommendation for Future Cycles:

_____

_____

Post-Cycle Testing Recommendations and Results:

_____

_____

Multiple Cycle Journaling Space

Cycle Number: _____ Cycle Date: _____

Notes:

_____

_____

_____

_____

_____

_____

_____

_____

_____

_____

_____

_____

_____

_____

_____

_____

_____

_____

_____

_____

Conclusion

Beautiful readers, I am so grateful to G-d and life for allowing me to walk this IVF journey. I learned so much from it, even though it was not easy. For me, it was an emotional time, a huge tumultuous storm of feelings, emotions, and moods. I went through IVF five times, but following this path gave me two amazing gifts, two wonderful girls.

It also gave me an angel, my Isabelle, who was stillborn at thirty-nine weeks, but even that event taught me so much and showed me that pain does not last forever. Thank you so much for allowing me to guide you with this planner during your cycle, and I hope it has helped you find the support and help you need. I encourage you to continue doing your best to shift your thoughts and actions to positive ones, to make your IVF journey pleasant and happy instead of stressful.

Wishing you love, light, and lots of baby dust,

Monica Bivas

PART VIII

GLOSSARY OF ACRONYMS AND TERMS

Glossary

2WW. Two-week wait (the slowest two weeks in the world).

A

ASAB. Antisperm antibodies. A very rare cause of infertility. Produced by both men or women. Actively kill sperm.

AF. Aunt Flo. A prudish way of saying *period*.

AHI. At-home insemination. DIY baby.

AI. Artificial insemination. Sophisticated turkey basting. Helps sperm get to their goal faster, easier, and more smoothly.

Assisted Hatching. A newer lab technique that was developed when fertility experts observed that embryos with a thin zona pellucida had a higher rate of implantation during IVF. With assisted hatching, an embryologist uses micromanipulation under a microscope to create a small hole in the zona pellucida to allow easier fertilization.

ATM. At the moment.

ART. Assisted reproductive technology, with a little or a lot of help from science.

AWOL. A woman on Lupron.

B

BA. Baby aspirin. Used during treatment to dilute the blood.

Babydust. Good wishes. (They mean well; just nod and smile.)

B/C. Because.

BeTa. Human chorionic gonadotropin (HCG) hormone pregnancy test.

Blast. Blastocyst. Day 5 fully developed embryo.

BBT. Basal body temperature. Used when charting your body temperature to determine when you ovulate or if you're pregnant.

BCP. Birth control pills. Helps regulate or control your cycle with the aim to getting you pregnant.

BD,BMS. Baby dance or baby-making sex. Good old-fashioned sex.

BF. Boyfriend or breastfed (but never both).

BFN. Big fat negative or "bloody fucking negative," if I really want to emphasize how shitty this result is.

BFP. Big fat positive, especially when emphasizing how frickin' amazing this result is.

BW. Blood work; a regular pain-in-the-arse-part of fertility treatment.

C

C#. Cycle number.

CB. Cycle buddy.

CGH. Comparative genomic hybridization (CGH). Also referred to as chromosomal microarray analysis (CMA) and array CGH (aCGH). A method of genetic testing.

CM. Cervical mucus. It sounds gross, but getting acquainted with your egg white discharge helps you detect when you're ovulating.

CP. Cervical positioning. Another way to detect where you are in your cycle.

CNM. Certified nurse midwife.

D

D&C. Dilation and curettage. Removal of a fetus (e.g., due to missed miscarriage).

Day 3 Test. Blood work and an ultrasound completed on the third day of a woman's cycle. Used to access reproductive potential.

Day 5 Test. Blood work and an ultrasound completed on the fifth day of a woman's cycle. Used to access reproductive potential.

DE. Donor eggs.

DIY. Do it yourself. Usually applies to crafts or projects.

DH. Dear/damn husband. All depending on what mood you're in.

DPO. Days post-ovulation.

DPR. Days post-retrieval.

DPT. Days post-transfer.

DW. Dear/darling/delightful/dazzling wife.

DX. Diagnosis.

E

E2. Estradiol, a type of oestrogen.

EDD. Estimated due date.

Embies. Embryos. One- to three-day fertilized eggs.

Endo. Endometriosis.

EPO. Evening primrose oil. Used for premenstrual syndrome (PMS), breast pain, endometriosis, and symptoms of menopause such as hot flashes.

EPT. Early pregnancy test. (We all do it.)

ER. Egg retrieval, surgical.

ET. Embryo transfer. The final step of IVF when embryos are placed into the uterus.

F

FET. Frozen embryo transfer.

FF. Fertility friend. (Everyone needs one of these.)

FHR. Fetal heart rate.

FP. Follicular phase. The first half of your menstrual cycle and the time it takes the ovary to release an egg.

FSH. Follicle-stimulating hormone, which stimulates the ovaries to create follicles. The synthetic version (e.g., Gonal F) is injected daily up until ovulation.

FTTA. Fertile thoughts to all from the baby dust family. (It's a nice sentiment, but sometimes feels a bit Disney in nature.)

FET. Frozen embryo transfer.

Follies. Follicles. The fluid-filled sacs on your ovaries that release your eggs.

Frosties. Frozen embryos.

FSH. Follicle-stimulating hormone.

G

GAL. Get a life. (Yeah, I'm trying.)

GFY. Good for you.

GIFT. Gamete intrafallopian transfer. The same as IVF, but with this method, fertilization happens inside the fallopian tubes, not the lab.

GnRH. Gonadotropin-releasing hormone. Also known as luteinizing hormone-releasing hormone (LHRH), responsible for the release of FSH and LH.

GP. General practitioner.

H

HCG. Human chorionic gonadotropin. A pregnancy hormone produced after implantation. The hormone most pregnancy tests detect.

HPT. Home pregnancy test.

HSC. Hysteroscopy. An internal scan through the cervix and uterus.

HTH. Hope that helps.

HX. Personal fertility background, not a fertility history lesson.

I

IAC. In any case.

ICI. Intracervical insemination. A cheaper, old-school procedure like IUI, but the sperm is placed near the cervix and not in the fallopian tubes.

ICSI. Intracytoplasmic sperm injection. Direct injection of the best sperm into the best egg.

ICBW. I could be wrong.

IDTT. I'll drink to that.

IF. Infertility. (It ain't easy getting knocked up.)

IME. In my experience.

IMO. In my opinion.

IUI. Intrauterine insemination. A form of AI. Sophisticated turkey-basting.

IVF. In vitro fertilization.

J

JIC. Just in case.

J/K. Just kidding.

JTYWLTK. Just thought you would like to know.

K

KUP. Keep us posted.

KWIM. Know what I mean.

L

LAP. Laparoscopy. A procedure where a camera is inserted through an incision to inspect or diagnose fertility problems.

LH. Luteinizing hormone. Secreted by the anterior pituitary gland, which stimulates ovulation.

LHRH. Luteinizing hormone-releasing hormone. Also known as gonadotropin-releasing hormone (GnRH). Responsible for the release of FSH and LH.

LMP. Last menstrual period, specifically the start date.

LO. Love Olympics. (Specifically sex, but you don't win a gold medal.)

LP. Luteal phase. From ovulation to menstruation, usually around twelve to fourteen days.

LSP. Low sperm count.

M

MC. Miscarriage.

MF. Male factor. Doctors specify the cause of infertility as male, female, or both.

M/S. Morning sickness.

Morula. A Day 4 embryo. The stage between embryo and blastocyst.

N

NAK. Nursing at keyboard.

NK. Natural killer cells. Lymphocytes in the immune system.

NP. No problem.

NRN. No reply necessary.

O

O, OV. Ovulation.

OB. Obstetrician.

OB-GYN. Obstetrician/Gynecologist.

OC. Oral contraceptives.

OD. Ovulatory dysfunction.

OHSS. Ovarian hyperstimulation syndrome, which can be triggered by using too many or too high a dose of certain medications. Doctors will not let you finish an IVF cycle if you have OHSS.

OPK. Ovulation predictor kit.

OPT. Ovulation predictor test.

OTC. Over-the-counter.

P

PCP. Primary care physician. Doctor.

PG. Pregnant. (Yes, please.)

PI. Primary infertility.

PID. Pelvic inflammatory disease.

PNV. Prenatal vitamin. (Our new BFF.)

POAS. Pee on a stick (when testing for ovulation and pregnancy).

PTL. Praise the Lord.

PUPO. Pregnant until proven otherwise. (Geez, do we need a lawyer for this?)

R

RE. Reproductive endocrinologist. Fertility doctor.

RPL. Recurrent pregnancy loss.

RX. Prescription.

S

SA. Semen analysis.

SBT. Sad but true.

SHG. SonoHSG. Sonohysterogram.

SI. Secondary infertility.

SITD. Still in the dark.

SIS. Saline injection sonogram.

SMEP. Sperm meets egg plan.

SO. Significant other.

STD. Sexually transmitted disease. (Fertility treatment requires regular testing.)

T

THX. Thanks.

TIME. Tears in my eyes.

IVF treatment may be the hardest thing you've ever done, but now you're not alone. Going through IVF treatment is simultaneously the easiest and hardest thing you'll ever do. Making the decision to go through treatment is an easy choice, but dealing with the emotions that emerge and keeping track of all the information can be daunting.

The IVF Planner offers guidance, information, and valuable advice to guide you through each aspect of your treatment. Detailed sections cover everything from the medical procedures you'll experience to coping with the emotions involved. Reduce your stress, connect with yourself, and set yourself up for a successful final outcome: a beautiful baby.

INDEX

A

able   viii, xiii

about   viii, xiv-xvi, 3-6, 9-12, 17, 40, 45, 50, 91-2, 96, 101, 117, 123

absorb   vii

accepting   vii

achieve   ix

acronyms   xvi, 135

ACRONYMS   135

across   xiv, xvi

actually   viii, 8

add   viii, 40

addresses   xv

adjustments   xii, 30, 45

advice   ix, xii-xiii, xvi, 96, 102, 115-16, 145

affect   viii, xiii, 12

after   vii-viii, x, 3-6, 12, 20, 50, 91-2, 96-7, 102, 140

After   vii-viii, x, 4-5, 12, 20

ago   vii, x

ahead   xiv, 11, 40, 92, 123

all   viii-ix, xi-xv, 3, 5, 8, 10, 12, 17, 31, 40, 45, 49, 75, 96-7, 138-9

All   138

allowing   vii-viii, 134

almost   vii, 49

already   vii-viii, xiii, 7, 41, 75, 101, 123

also   vii-x, xiii-xv, 3-11, 17-18, 31, 45, 49-50, 75, 91-2, 96-7, 101, 117-18, 123, 134, 137

always   ix, 3, 7-8, 10, 49, 117

Always   ix

am   viii, x-xi, 11, 92, 134

amazing   viii-ix, 49, 75, 134, 137

amount   ix, 9, 31-2, 37, 91

an   vii-ix, xiii-xiv, xvi, 3-8, 10-12, 39-40, 44, 49, 74, 92, 101, 134, 136, 138-41, 143

and   vii-xvi, 2-12, 16-18, 20-1, 30-1, 39-41, 44-6, 49-50, 73-5, 91-2, 96-7, 100-2, 117-18, 122-4, 134-40

AND   16, 24-5, 30, 39, 49, 73, 100, 122-3, 135

another   vii, 3, 92, 97, 117, 123, 138

answer   xiii, 17, 26-7

answers   viii, 17

anticipated   xiii

any   xiii, 2, 6-7, 9-10, 18, 31, 40-1, 45, 75, 101-2, 140

applicable   xii, xiv, 30

apply   xiv

appointments   xii, 2, 49

approach   viii-ix

are   vii-x, xii-xvi, 2-11, 17, 30-1, 39-40, 44-6, 49-50, 74-5, 91-2, 96, 101, 117, 123, 138-9

articles   xii

as   vii-x, xiii-xiv, xvi, 2-5, 7-9, 17-18, 30-1, 39-40, 74-5, 91, 96, 101, 117-18, 139-40, 142

aspects   viii, xv

Assisted   xiv, 5, 11, 117, 136

assists   xv

assumes   xiii

depending   xiii, 5-6, 39, 46, 138

depends   xiii, 3, 6, 30, 75

describes   xiv

designed   xv, 17

detail   xiv, 7

detailed   xiv, 11-12, 31, 40, 145

details   xiv, 18, 31-2, 34-5, 49-51,
     98-9, 119-21

diagnosis   xiii-xiv, 5, 9-13, 91, 138

Diagnosis   10-11, 13, 138

did   vii, 75, 97

differ   xiii

different   viii, xii-xiv, 2, 75

difficult   vii, 9-11, 44, 49, 74

directly   xiii

disciplined   ix

discovery   xiii

divided   xiv, 2, 12, 50

do   viii, xiii-xiv, 3-5, 8-10, 39-40,
     44-5, 50, 74-5, 92, 96, 123,
     138-9, 143, 145

doctor   viii, 24-5, 143

document   viii, 18

doesn   xii, 4

doing   viii, 10, 39, 134

don   xii-xiii, 11, 17, 39-40, 45-6,
     97, 142

Don   17, 97

done   x, xiii, 3-6, 145

donor   xii, 138

double   vii

doubts   xiii

down   xv, 40, 44-5, 102

due   vii, 92, 96, 138

during   viii, x, xii, xiv-xv, 3-4, 6, 8,
     17-18, 31, 44-5, 49-50, 92,
     96-7, 101-2, 136

E

each   viii-ix, xii-xv, 3-4, 6, 30-1,
     40, 123, 145

Each   viii, xiv, 6

ease   xii, xv, 74, 96

easier   xvi, 2, 45, 49-50, 101,
     123, 136

easily   viii

easy   xv, 11-12, 44, 96, 101, 134,
     141, 145

effort   ix, 10

egg   xv, 2-5, 7, 9, 50, 67, 69-70,
     137, 139, 141, 144

eggs   xii, 2-5, 9, 50, 70, 138-9

eight   xiv, 44

Eliyah   viii, x

emails   xv

embryo   xii, xv, 2, 5-9, 12, 14,
     21, 50, 70-2, 74-5, 91, 137,
     139, 142

Embryo   5, 14, 21, 50, 70-2,
     75, 139

emotional   viii, x, xiv-xv, 94, 96,
     101, 134

EMOTIONAL   101

emotions   vii-viii, xii, xv, 10, 44-5,
     101, 134, 145

end   ix, xii-xiii, xv, 6, 8, 18, 45, 91-
     2, 97

ended   vii

endless   xii

Endocrinologist   viii, xiii, 143

endometriosis   vii, x, 9, 139

enough   xiv, 44

ER   xv, 139

especially   xii, 4, 7, 45, 75, 137

ET   xv, 139

even   vii-xii, xiv, 6-8, 10-11, 31, 45,
     91-2, 96, 101, 123, 134

every   vii, xii-xiii, 2-3, 9, 17, 40, 96

Every   vii, xii, 2, 17

evolving   xiii

exactly   viii, 31, 92, 97

exhaustive   xvi

expected vii, 11, 96

expense xv, 36, 40

expensive xii, 5

experience ix, xiii, 4, 7, 96, 101, 141, 145

experiences vii-viii

explanation xiv, 11

explore xv

extremely vii, 9, 44

F

Fat vii, xiii, 91, 137

feedback xii

feel ix-x, xiv, 4, 45, 92

feelings vii-viii, 18, 44-5, 101, 103-14, 123, 134

fertility vii-viii, x, 7, 9, 11, 39, 41, 92, 94, 96, 117, 136-7, 139-41, 143-4

Fertilization 5, 50

FET xvi, 122-3, 139

few xii, 2-3, 6-7, 10, 39

fill xv, 12, 17, 31, 46, 50, 91, 96-7

finances xiii, xv, 29-31

FINANCES 29-30

financial xii, xiv-xv, 30-1

financing xv

find viii-ix, xv, 5, 9, 11, 31, 39-40, 49-50, 92, 96, 117, 123, 134

firestorm xiv

first vii-viii, x, 11, 41, 45, 50, 91, 96-7, 139

five vii, 2, 4-5, 39, 50, 74, 134

focus vii, ix, xii, 10, 45, 74, 96, 101, 123

focused ix

for ix-xvi, 2-7, 9-12, 17, 30-2, 39-41, 44-5, 49-51, 91-2, 96-8, 117, 123-4, 134, 139-40, 142-3

FOR 10, 91

found xii, 49, 74

fourth vii

free x, xv, 117

from vii-x, xiii, 2-4, 7, 30, 40, 75, 96-7, 117, 134, 136, 139, 142, 145

full xiii, 6-8

G

GATHERING 117

general xii, xiv, 91, 124, 126, 128, 130, 132, 140

get xi, xiii-xiv, 5, 39, 45, 91, 97, 117, 123, 136, 140

Get xiii, 140

getting vii, 97, 137, 141

girl vii, 96

give xiii, 11, 40, 49

given ix, 3, 6

glossary xiv, xvi, 135-6

Glossary xiv, xvi

GLOSSARY 135-6

go ix-x, xiii-xiv, xvi, 6, 39, 45, 92, 96-7, 102, 117, 123, 145

goal viii, 136

going vii-viii, xii, 10-11, 44-5, 49, 117, 145

gone xiii-xiv

good ix, 6, 8, 12, 40-1, 75, 123, 136-7, 140

Google xiii

greater vii

group xv, 11, 92, 117

groups xvi, 11, 17, 92, 96, 117-18

Growth 5, 70

guidance ix, 4, 40, 145

guide ix, 7, 39-40, 92, 134, 145

GUIDE 39

H

half viii, x, 139

handle   vii, xii, xv, 101-2, 117
handling   xv
has   vii, xiii, 6-7, 31, 39, 50,
    96, 134
have   vii-xiv, 2-4, 6, 8, 11-12, 18,
    30-1, 39-41, 44-5, 49, 74, 92,
    117, 123, 143
having   vii-viii, xv, 3, 8, 45, 91
healthy   vii, xiii, 8, 11, 44, 74, 96
heart   ix-x, 96, 139
help   vii-ix, xii, xiv-xv, 3, 5-6, 8, 11-
    12, 17, 30-1, 44-5, 74-5, 91,
    101-2, 123, 134
helped   vii-viii, x-xi, 134
helpful   xii, xv, 45, 117
helps   ix, xv, 31, 75, 101, 117, 136-
    7, 140
her   vii, ix, xiii, 2, 39, 96
Here   xv, 7, 10, 12, 30, 39, 74
him   ix, 39
his   xiii, 2
hope   ix, 5, 101, 134, 140
hours   ix, 3, 20, 22-3
However   vii-viii, xiii-xiv, 3-5, 49
husband   viii, x, 138

I

if   ix, xii-xiv, xvi, 3-4, 6-9, 11, 30-1,
    39-41, 44-5, 74-5, 91-2, 96-
    7, 101, 123, 137
If   xiii, 4, 6, 11, 30, 39-41, 44-5,
    74-5, 92, 96-7, 101
II   xv, 16
III   xv, 29
immediately   vii, 123
in   vii-xvi, 2-11, 17-18, 30-1, 40-
    1, 44-5, 49-50, 74-5, 91-2,
    96-7, 101, 117-18, 123, 136-
    42, 144

In   vii, ix, xiii-xv, 2, 4, 7, 11, 30-1,
    45, 50, 74-5, 96, 117, 123,
    140-1
included   xiii, 31-2, 50, 74
includes   xii, 2, 10, 18, 31, 49, 97
including   vii, 31
increases   xiii, 3, 7
individual   viii
infertility   xiii-xiv, 9, 117, 136, 141-4
information   vii, ix, xii-xvi, 9-12,
    17-18, 20-1, 31-2, 40, 45, 50,
    67, 69-71, 91, 96, 145
insensitive   xiii
insurance   xii, xv, 30-5, 41, 92
interact   xiii, 17, 117
into   ix-x, xiv, 2, 4, 6, 44, 49-50,
    139, 141
INTRODUCTION   xii
investment   xii
involve   xii
involved   viii, xiv, 18, 145
is   vii-x, xii-xvi, 2-12, 17-18, 30-1,
    39-40, 44-5, 49-50, 74-5,
    91-2, 96-7, 101, 117, 137,
    139-41
Isabelle   vi, x, 134
issues   vii-viii, 2, 9, 96
it   vii-x, xii-xvi, 2-12, 17-18, 30-1,
    39-40, 44-5, 49-50, 74-5, 91,
    96-7, 101-2, 117, 134, 137-9
It   vii, ix, xii-xvi, 3, 7-8, 12, 18,
    30-1, 39-40, 45, 50, 91, 96,
    101, 134
its   xv, 6, 17, 44
itself   vii, xv, 8, 10
IV   xv, 43
IVF   vi-159, 161, 163, 165, 167

J

joining   xv, 11

we   ix-x, xvi, 8, 11, 44, 74-5, 91,
      96, 123, 139, 143
We   ix, 75, 91, 96, 139
website   xiv, 11, 22-5, 32, 74,
      92, 117
websites   xii, 117-18
week   xv, 7-8, 74, 96, 136
WEEK   74
weeks   vii, 2-3, 44, 91, 134, 136
well   xvi, 8, 10, 18, 30, 74, 97, 136
were   vii, x-xi, 4, 50, 75, 96
what   vii-viii, x, xii-xiii, xvi, 9-11,
      17, 31, 40, 45, 91-2, 123,
      138, 141
What   xii-xiii
when   ix-x, xiv, 4, 6-12, 30-1, 39-
      40, 44-5, 97, 123, 136-7,
      139, 143
where   xi, xiii, 2, 17, 45, 49, 123,
      138, 141
whether   xiv, 5, 30-1, 39-40, 75,
      102, 123
which   xii, xiv, 3-4, 6-12, 17-18,
      30-1, 45, 49-50, 91, 139,
      141, 143
who   viii-ix, xi, 4, 9, 11, 17, 30-1,
      49, 117, 134
why   xiii-xiv, 11-12, 44, 91, 101
Why   xiv
will   viii-ix, xii-xv, 2-7, 9, 12, 17, 30-
      1, 39-41, 45, 49-50, 96-7,
      101, 123, 143
with   vii-x, xii-xvi, 3-9, 11-12, 17,
      31, 44-6, 49-50, 74-5, 92,
      96, 101, 117, 136-7, 145
With   vii-ix, 136
WITH   96
without   x, 96
woman   xii, 2, 101, 136, 138
women   viii-ix, xi-xiii, xvi, 2, 4, 7-9,
      11, 39, 45, 96, 117, 136

wonderful   xiii, 74, 134
world   ix, 117, 136
worth   ix, 5
would   vii, x, xiv, 141
write   ix, xii, 31, 102
writing   xv, 45, 101, 123
written   xvi
wrong   xiii, 141
www   xiv, 11, 40, 74, 92, 117

Y

year   vii, x, 40
years   x, 7, 11, 39
Yes   xii, 143
you   viii-xvi, 2-12, 17-18, 30-1, 39-
      41, 44-6, 49-50, 74-5, 91-2,
      96-7, 101-2, 117-18, 123,
      134, 137-8
You   x, xii-xiii, 2-4, 6-7, 11, 17, 40,
      49-50, 92, 97, 117-18, 123
your   viii-x, xii-xv, 2-12, 17-18, 30-
      1, 39-41, 44-6, 49-50, 73-5,
      91-2, 96-7, 101-2, 117-18,
      123, 137-9
Your   x, xii-xiii, xv, 2-4, 8, 10-11,
      40, 45
YOUR   17, 30, 73, 91, 117
yourself   ix, xii, 49, 74, 96-7, 117,
      138, 145

CPSIA information can be obtained
at www.ICGtesting.com
Printed in the USA
FSHW021047161118
53842FS